CW00348725

Bowles's Universal Display of the Naval Flags of all Nations in the World. = Bowles's vue Universelle des Pavillons Marine

BOWLES's
UNIVERSAL DISPLAY
OF THE
NAVAL FLAGS
of all
NATIONS
in the
WORLD.

* * *

Printed for the Proprietors,

BOWLES & CARVER,

N°69 in St Paul's Church Yard,

LONDON

BOWLES's
VUE UNIVERSELLE DES
PAVILLONS MARINE
dans touts les PARTIES du
MONDE.

* * *

Imprimée pour les Proprietaires,

BOWLES & CARVER,

No 69 St Paul's Church Yard

a LONDRE

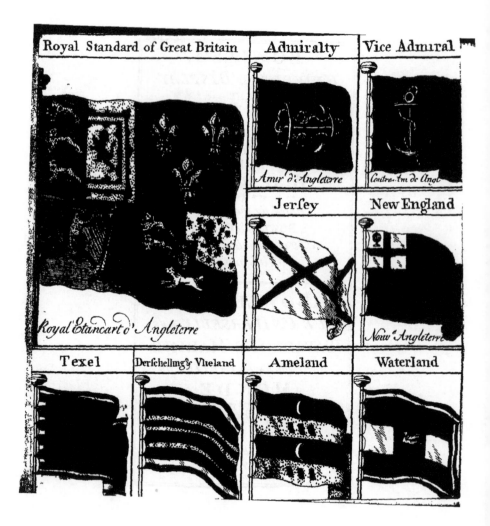

Royal Standard of Great Britain | Admiralty | Vice Admiral

Royal Etancart o' Angleterre | *Amir d'Angleterre* | *Contre Am de Angl*

Jersey | New England

Nouv Angleterre

Texel | Derschelling & Vlieland | Ameland | Waterland

Red Enfign	White Enfign	Blue Enfign	Union Jack
Nouv.e Union de la grand Bretagne	*Anglois particulier*		*du Jac d' Angleterre*
Guine a Jack	States General	Princes Flag	Double Prince
du Jac pour Guinee en Angletere	*Etal. Gener.r d.es Provinces Vnies*	*de l'Etat dit du Prince*	*le Double du Prince*
Zeland	Middleburgh	Middleburgh Jack	Vliffinge Jack
	Middelbourg	*du Poupe de Middelbourg*	

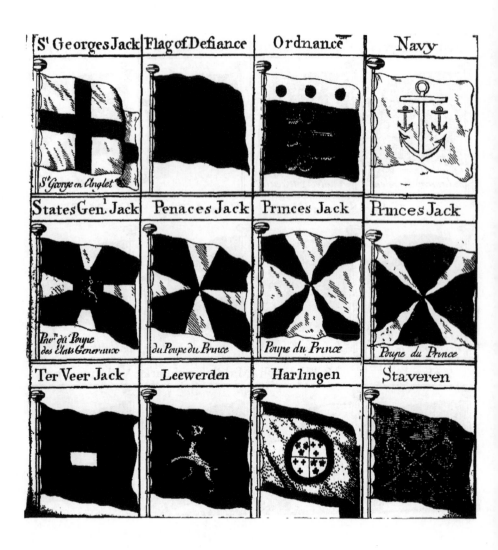

S.t Georges Jack	Flag of Defiance	Ordnance	Navy
S.t George en Anglet			
States Gen.l Jack	Penaces Jack	Princes Jack	Princes Jack
Pav.on du Poupe des Etats Generaux	du Poupe du Prince	Poupe du Prince	Poupe du Prince
Ter Veer Jack	Leewerden	Harlingen	Staveren

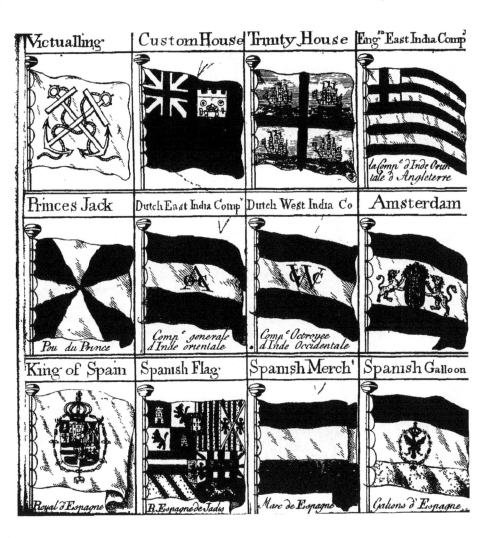

Victualling	Custom House	Trinity House	Eng.ᵗᵈ East India Comp
			la Comp.ᵉ d'Inde Orien tale d'Angleterre
Princes Jack	Dutch East India Comp.ʸ	Dutch West India Co	Amsterdam
Pou du Prince	Comp.ᵉ generale d'Inde orientale	Comp.ᵉ Octroyee d'Inde Occidentale	
King of Spain	Spanish Flag	Spanish Merch.ᵗ	Spanish Galloon
Royal d'Espagne	R. Espagne de Jades	Marc de Espagne	Galions d'Espagne

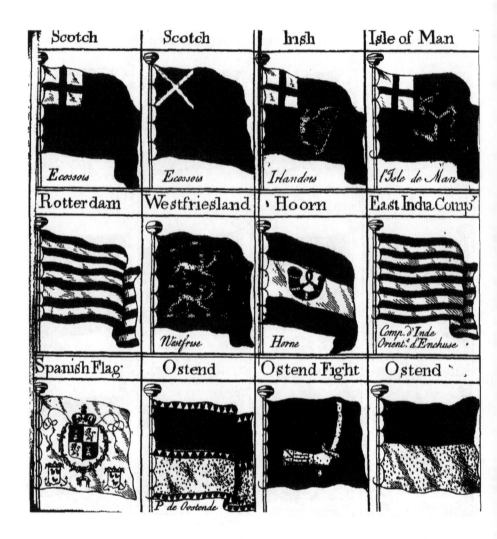

Scotch	Scotch	Irish	Isle of Man
Ecossois	*Ecossois*	*Irlandois*	*l'Isle de Man*
Rotterdam	Westfriesland	Hoorn	East India Comp.ᵞ
	Westfrise	*Horne*	*Comp. d'Inde Orient.ᵉ d'Enchuse*
Spanish Flag	Ostend	Ostend Fight	Ostend
	P. de Oostende		

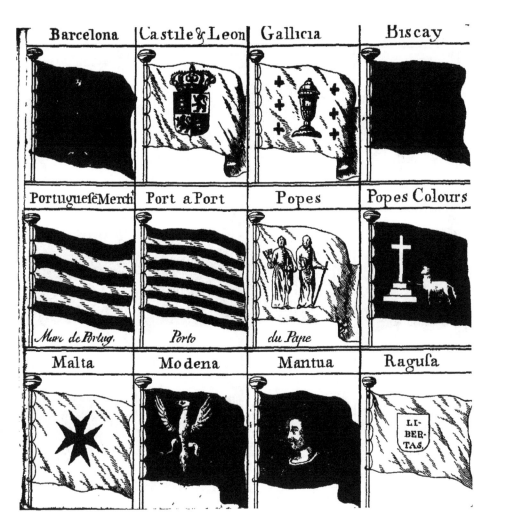

Barcelona	Castile & Leon	Gallicia	Biscay
Portuguese Merch	Port a Port	Popes	Popes Colours
Marc de Portug.	*Porto*	*du Pape*	
Malta	Modena	Mantua	Ragusa

LI-
BER-
TAS.

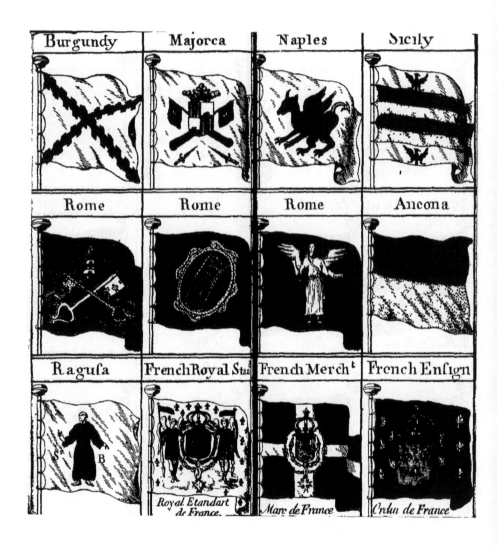

Burgundy	Majorca	Naples	Sicily
Rome	Rome	Rome	Ancona
Ragusa	French Royal Stan	French Merch.t	French Ensign
	Royal Etandart de France.	Marc de France	Ordm de France

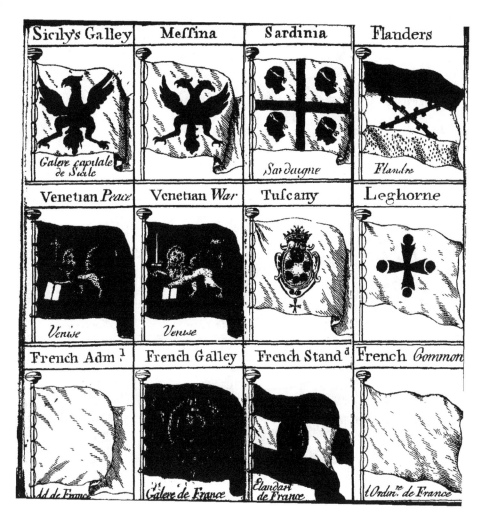

Sicily's Galley	Meſſina	Sardinia	Flanders
Galere capitale de Sicile		Sardaigne	Flandre

Venetian *Peace*	Venetian *War*	Tuſcany	Leghorne
Venise	Venise		

French Adm.ˡ	French Galley	French Stand.ᵈ	French *Common*
Ad de France	Galere de France	Etandart de France	l Ordin.ʳᵉ de France

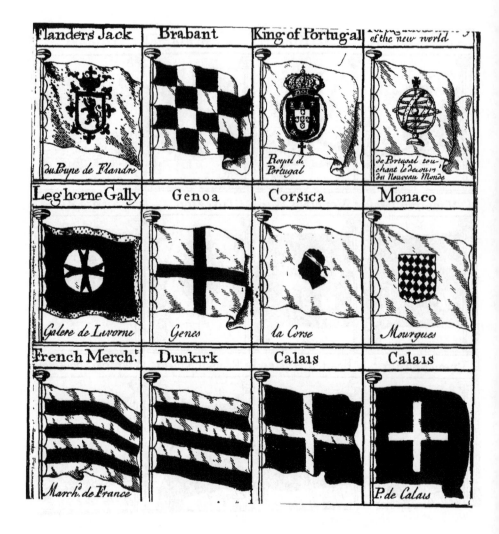

Flanders Jack	Brabant	King of Portugal	...of the new world
du Pape de Flandre		Royal de Portugal	de Portugal touchant le devoir du Nouveau Monde
Leghorne Gally	Genoa	Corsica	Monaco
Galere de Livorne	Genes	la Corse	Mourgues
French Merch.t	Dunkirk	Calais	Calais
March.o de France			P. de Calais

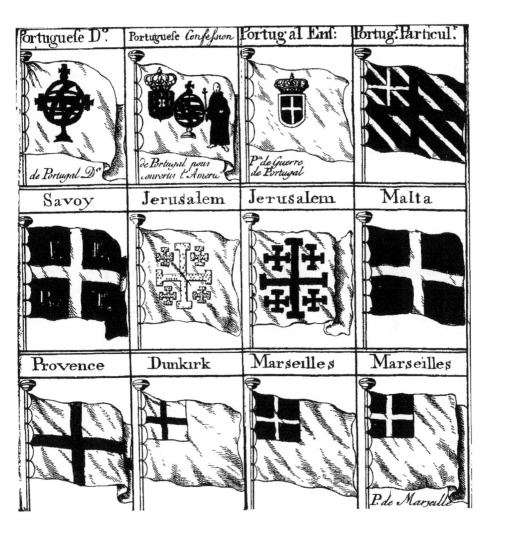

Portuguefe Dº.	Portuguefe *Confeffion*	Portug:al Enf:	Portug:Particul.ᵉ
de Portugal Dº.	*de Portugal pour convertir l'Ameriᵠ*	Pⁿ *de Guerre de Portugal*	
Savoy	Jerusalem	Jerusalem	Malta
Provence	Dunkirk	Marseilles	Marseilles

P. de Marseille

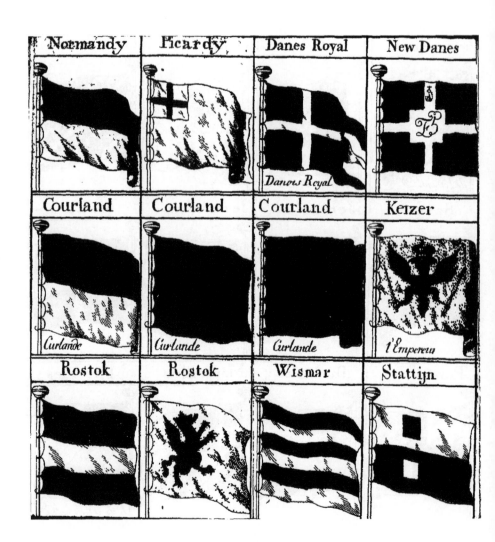

Normandy	Picardy	Danes Royal	New Danes
Courland	Courland	Courland	Keizer
Rostok	Rostok	Wismar	Stattijn

Danes Royal

Curlande   Curlande   Curlande   l'Empereu

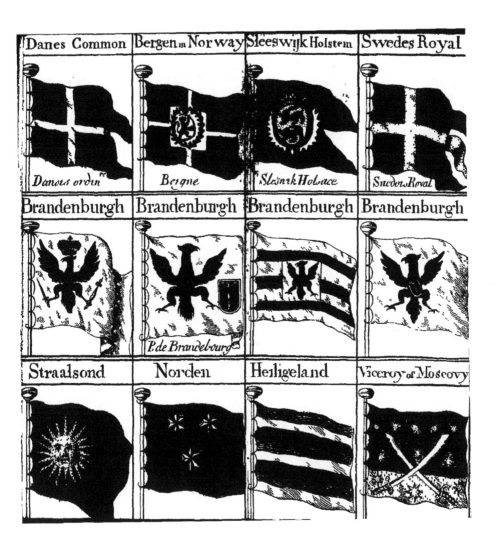

Danes Common	Bergen in Norway	Sleeswijk Holstein	Swedes Royal
Danes ordin.	*Bergne*	*Slesnik Holsace*	*Suedois Roval*
Brandenburgh	Brandenburgh	Brandenburgh	Brandenburgh
	P. de Brandebourg		
Straalsond	Norden	Heiligeland	Viceroy of Moscovy

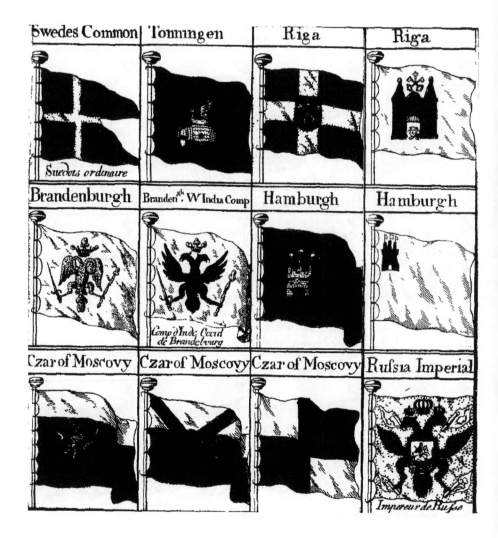

Swedes Common	Tonningen	Riga	Riga
Suedois ordinaire			
Brandenburgh	Branden^{gh}. W India Comp	Hamburgh	Hamburgh
	Comp d'Inde Occid de Brandebourg		
Czar of Moscovy	Czar of Moscovy	Czar of Moscovy	Russia Imperial
			Impereur de Russe

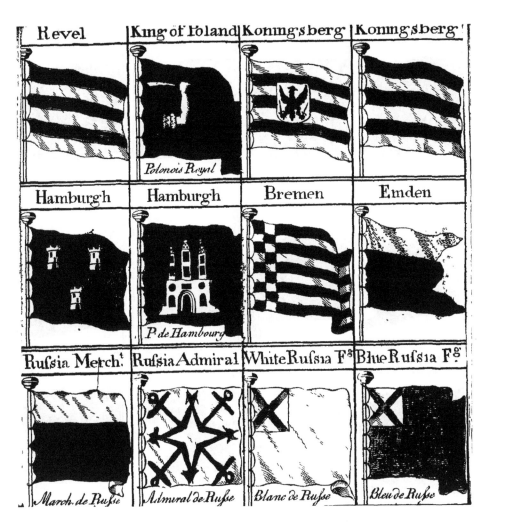

Revel	King of Poland	Konnigsberg	Konnigsberg
	Polonois Royal		
Hamburgh	Hamburgh	Bremen	Emden
	P. de Hambourg		
Russia Merch.ᵗ	Russia Admiral	White Russia Fˢ	Blue Russia Fˢ
March. de Russie	*Admiral de Russie*	*Blanc de Russie*	*Bleu de Russie*

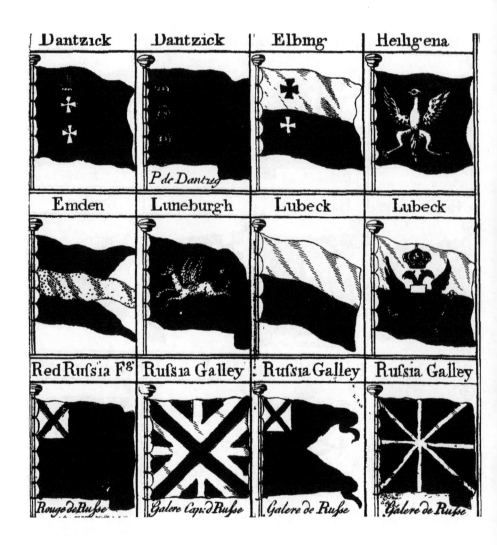

Dantzick	Dantzick	Elbing	Heiligena
	P de Dantzig		
Emden	Luneburgh	Lubeck	Lubeck
Red Russia Fg	Russia Galley	Russia Galley	Russia Galley
Rouge de Russe	*Galere Cap:d'Russe*	*Galere de Russe*	*Galere de Russe*

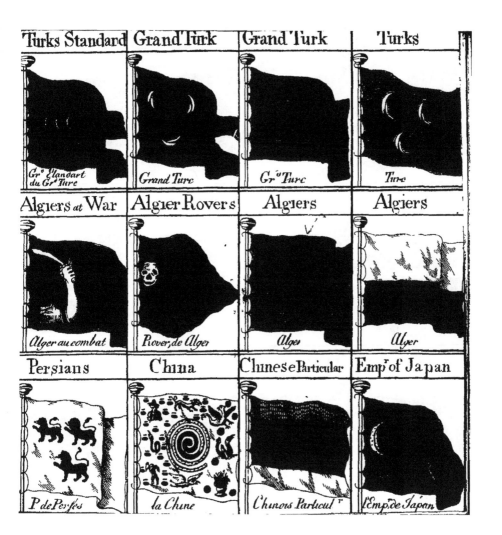

Turks Standard	Grand Turk	Grand Turk	Turks
Gr.ᵈ Etandart du Gr.ᵈ Turc	Grand Turc	Gr.ᵈ Turc	Turc
Algiers *at* War	Algier Rovers	Algiers	Algiers
Alger au combat	Rover de Alger	Alger	Alger
Persians	China	Chinese Particular	Emp.ʳ of Japan
P. de Perses	la Chine	Chinois Particul.ʳ	l'Emp.ʳ de Japan

Turks	Turks Galley	Turks Galley	Constantinople
Turc	*Galere Turque*	*Galere Turque*	
Algiers	Tetuan	Sangrian	Mamelik
Alger			
Emp.r of Tartarys	Tartary	Moores	Moores
l'Emp.r de Tartarie		*Mores*	

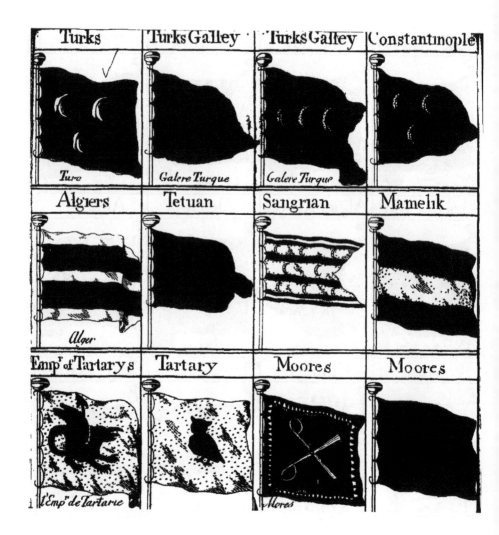

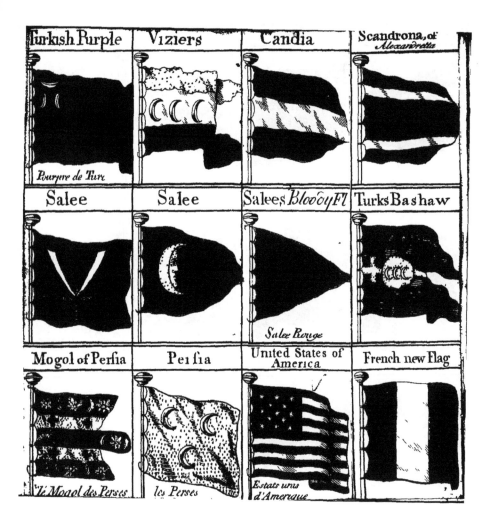

Turkish Purple | Viziers | Candia | Scandrona, or Alexandretta
Pourpre de Turc | | |
Salee | Salee | Salees Bloody Fl | Turks Bashaw
| | Salee Rouge |
Mogol of Persia | Persia | United States of America | French new Flag
Le Mogol des Perses | les Perses | Estats unis d'Amerique |

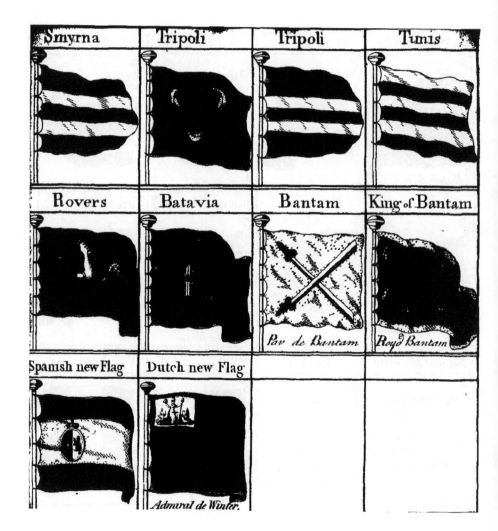

Smyrna	Tripoli	Tripoli	Tunis
Rovers	Batavia	Bantam	King of Bantam
		Pav de Bantam	*Roy.d Bantam*
Spanish new Flag	Dutch new Flag		
	Admiral de Winter.		

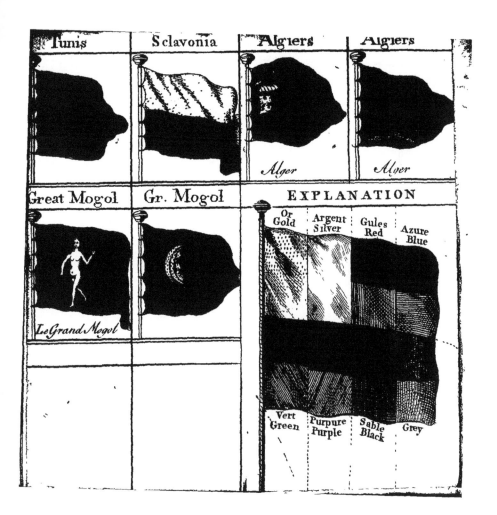

Tunis	Sclavonia	Algiers	Algiers
		Alger	*Alger*

Great Mogol	Gr. Mogol	EXPLANATION
Le Grand Mogol		

EXPLANATION

Or Gold   Argent Silver   Gules Red   Azure Blue

Vert Green   Purpure Purple   Sable Black   Grey

Lightning Source UK Ltd.
Milton Keynes UK
UKHW022335060223
416579UK00001B/4